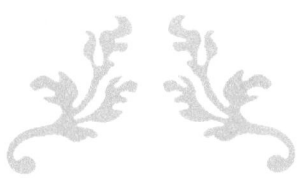

SOMEBODY GRAB THAT TURKEY BUZZARD! WE GOTS TO FIX DINNER!

Musings of a tortured Mind

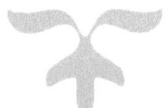

Angela Luck

And she said, "One day, I'll be beautiful, and you'll want me. But I won't be there."

Turkey Buzzard *Angela Luck*

Musings Series Book 1

ISBN: 9781726624152

Independently published through Amazon

First Edition: November 2018

Turkey Buzzard   *Angela Luck*

Preamble

In order to learn, you have to make a few mistakes. No-one is perfect. Least of all, me. I've managed to mess up too many marriages. That's why I won't do it again. If I'm wrong, God forgive me. I just can't do it anymore. I want to be happy and I want a man my age in my life but I don't want to burden him with paying for a divorce I should have gotten years ago and never bothered with because I didn't care.

When I actually did care enough to try, I got shafted by a shyster and then cheated on by the man I cared enough to maybe have married. So why bother now? Time will tell.

This journal entry is from October 7, 2017.

Life changes and I'm in hopes that writing some of my life and experiences, along with some of my musings in journal entries, will help others to find their way in this ever-changing life where so many have faltered along the wayside. I pray every day that my gift will be to touch another enough to make a difference.

Turkey Buzzard   *Angela Luck*

If perchance I make you smile, I make you laugh, or I help you understand and make a change for the better in your life,

then my life has been worthwhile. I've always heard that if you hide your light under a barrel it will never help anyone find the way. Maybe my light will shine and find someone's end of their tunnel.

So, without any more rabble and rigmarole, let's get this party started, shall we?

Bright blessings and God Bless!

Turkey Buzzard   Angela Luck

I started to start writing a few times before now I'm going to try to make myself do what I should have done. First off, I gotta tell you the God's Honest Down and Dirty Truth. If it shocks you, then it does. If not, then that's ok, too. I have to tell you the truth. I love you to death. I've said it before out loud to you, but I somehow don't even think you heard it or maybe you thought I was a little bit nutty, which I am, but not when it comes to my heart. I ramble on, but the truth is, I've thought about this for a while now and I can't seem to put it down.

Something you did sorta hurt my heart to tell the truth. I know it's how you feel, but it still hurt. When you wrote that on Facebook about no wife, no kids, no worries, it stung, it really did. Not like I was hoping you'd ask to marry me, because that's the furthest thing from my mind right now, to be honest. Yes, I'm female and yes, I won't lie, most of the time women want to get married, but I can't even begin to think about something like that right now. But truthfully, all I really want is what you've already given me in a sense. And whether either of us admit it or not, we kind of have a commitment. I'd like to hear it come from your lips, but that's immaterial, too, to be honest.

I really don't know why I'm even writing this, because everything I'm saying in this little (little?) letter is things that we've either already discussed or things that are just understood. Maybe I'm doing it to remind myself of the fact.

And why would I be reminding myself? This is so hilarious, I can just barely keep from laughing myself. Someone came along who actually asked me to marry him while we were on hiatus from one another. I've thought about it, which mostly was thinking how totally ridiculous it really is, but still I thought. It was, for the most part, someone who is more in love with being in love and who is captivated by the thought of marriage, but for all the wrong reasons. Marriage is something that, if it's right, it's beautiful and yet, there's always something that you have to handle together. It's not just having the same sexual partner for the rest of your life, but also having the person who is your best friend there with you for the rest of your life, too. And if that's not the case and you can't talk or share or work together, then it's not right and it never will be. I guess that's why I think marriage is ridiculous right now. And I don't know if I'll ever change my mind about it, either.

The dissertation on marriage was more for my own benefit than for yours, by the way. It was just something I needed to air out. Plus, honestly, this letter will probably never make it past right here, so it doesn't matter anyhow.

I have other things that I feel I have to say to you, but they're so jumbled up inside my head that I simply can't begin to say them in a logical sequence. I guess that's another reason I write.

All I did the whole time we didn't talk was think about you and texting you and being with you. It's silly, I know, but it's so true. I missed you pretty badly. I guess that's why I sorta let this other person talk to me, too. To keep from missing you so badly because I thought it would be good for us just to not talk for a day and see if my feelings or yours changed. I'm sure about mine, now. Not so sure about yours. And I

Turkey Buzzard   *Angela Luck*

guess I'll just about always be partially in the dark about how you feel because you've been hurt so bad, you've got a hole bigger than mine in your heart. And I know what that's like because I keep trying to cover mine up, but somehow the damn thing starts getting torn back apart again.

Feeling like I feel about you only makes it worse sometimes, too. Because love is a scary thing. Especially when you have had someone rip your heart out by the roots and kick it around for a while. It honestly scares me to death missing you like I do because I know that's part of being in love with you…and yes, I said IN love…and yes, it scares the holy bejesus out of me, too. I know you would never hurt me knowingly. But there too, I guess I do have a streak of a coward in me. Or maybe it's the lack thereof. I don't want to be hurt, but I was willing to jump in with you. Whether you want me or not. And I know you WANT me…but I guess I mean if you WANT me like a girlfriend or if you want something else. Seriously, I'd like to know for sure. Anyway, I think I'm finished with this for now. I may write more when I can think straight again.

My sons have me off on a money tangent now. I do love you. I know I could love you more than I do and eventually I could love you more than I've ever love anyone before. And I can help you fix the hole in your heart if you'll do the same for me.

This was written in 2011 to someone I should have been with and failed

miserably. He died without ever reading it or knowing that I'd love him until the day I die. He never saw that I went off the chain when he was killed or knew that I still to this day feel guilty over his death, because I feel that if we had been together, he wouldn't have been killed by the bastard who killed him.

While I may have a lackadaisical attitude toward death in many ways, my thoughts on his death at long and crippling. I'll never learn not to blame myself for the lost love of a man so sweet that he did all he could to make my life better and I allowed an asshole who I'd been with longer to come back into my life and tear us apart.

Maybe, just maybe, it was happening all the time. Maybe I just didn't see it. Maybe I really was as sweet and innocent as I pretended to be. And as naïve. Every time I think about this, it makes me feel more and more stupid.

It was, for much of my adult life, my dubious blessing to have had a nice set of legs, an ample busom, and somewhat charming personality. I say or write this with a tongue-in-cheek, knowing full well that all of the above criteria are subjective. However, I, myself, only played upon the entire thing to begin with.

Having been an obese child, I could only see myself as such an adult, too. And, for a good portion of my life, it was quite true. In my thought, no man actually looks at a fat chick.

So, in the interest of being flamboyant, I developed my own style. I dress in bright colors, short shorts, jackets to call attention to it all. I had enough see-thru shirts to float a battleship, that I wore tanks or colored bras under. Still, I never noticed anyone paying much attention. Heck, I got more attention from women than from men.

Then there was this year.

When I first saw the look, I thought I surely had mistaken it.

I'd been talking to the guy online, helping him with his grief. His wife of 20+ years had died only a few months earlier and I'd been recruited by a friend to help him. It was something that was "right up my alley" so to speak. I was good at dealing with others' problems.

I was a perfect counselor, I thought.

A few months in, he'd wanted to meet me in person and offered to drive me to a doctors' appointment. It seemed harmless enough. As did he.

We talked on the way to me doctor's office. As he was helping me out of the car, I caught in the corner of my eye, a look I'd never seen before in anyone. And it was so quickly gone, I chose to think I'd been wrong.

On his face, I did see it. I wish I'd believed I had, then. It would have saved me from a lot of stress and heartache.

That look should have given me a clue.

I was too dumb. And it would have kept me away from something that eventually dug an even bigger hole in my soul than was already there.

His eyes were hooded, piercing. He gazed up and down my body like he was a starving man gazing at a piece of meat. That look in his eyes that day was only for a second, but I know, now, what it was. It was pure carnal lust.

That look, I saw many more times after I consented to go out with him. But there was so much more there, behind that look of lust. There also was the driving desire to possess, (not love, not enjoy, or care for) to totally own every fiber of my being.

It was the last look I can remember from that last day I spent with him, too. It was the last look I can remember from him on that last night I spent with him. It was the night I told him no, because I was too tired.

I'd worked 10 hours at work that day. I drove for an hour and a half to get to his house. We'd stayed up visiting with his family and more had come in and left, too. It was nearly 2am. I'd been up since 4am the previous day.

He made his move. I said no and explained that I was very dead tired. He didn't want to take "no" for an answer. And there was that look again. He tried to force me.

Turkey Buzzard   *Angela Luck*

For all intents and purposes, right there, I was through. I knew once I'd had some sleep (unless he raped me), I was going to head home tomorrow and I wasn't coming back for a very long time, if ever.

I was going to leave in the morning and maybe never come back at all.

I knew if he did force himself on me, I'd wait for him to go to sleep, hit him with something and run.

And you know something? I know for a fact that I'm no Madonna or Marilyn Monroe, but I know there's *NOTHING* that special about me. But, since then, I've seen "that look" twice.

I don't like it.

When I do see it, I tend to weigh my options very carefully.

Both times have ended with me back on the outside. Far as I'm concerned, outside might me the best place to be in that case.

Turkey Buzzard   *Angela Luck*

I am the silver in that dark cloud.

I am the lightening in the dark sky.

I am the fire that can't be vanquished.

I am the vision that rides on high.

I am the passion that has no end.

I am the storm that arrives without warning.

I am the heart that loves without qualm.

I am the truth that you'll hear in the morning.

I am the blackest of black heart revenge.

I am protection for love of my friends.

I am a story with so many turns.

I am the Love and a love without ends.

I am who I am

I am who I'll be

I love with all fury

Wish someone would love me.

®︎ Angela Luck 2018

April 9, 2017

Thoughts in the shower: No, I am not thin or shapely. Some may not even call me beautiful.

No, I am not young anymore, but my heart sings just the same as a young girl's does when the man she loves holds her in his arms and softly says, 'I love you.'

No, I am not average either. Nor am I ladylike or helpless. But I am overjoyed and so very delighted when those who love me step up when I need them, be it morally, mentally, or physically.

I am not a fragile flower, but I do have moments that I will and do cry. Respect that, just as I respect it in all of you. Sometimes tears are NOT a sign of weakness, but of heart.

I am me. And for all that I am, to me, and to those who are privy to see beyond the veil, I am one thing and that is EXCEPTIONAL.

Turkey Buzzard   Angela Luck

June 17, 2017

A lot of people may see me as a lot of things but one thing I'm not is a drama queen. Never have been and never will be. I despise drama in every way. My age and my mental state have made me hate it all the more. I try to stay out of situations that will bring more stress into my already stressful life. Dealing with too much stress isn't conductive to prime mental health for me. And in order to keep my little family together and strong, I need to be strong. This is a sounding board for me sometimes and hopefully my friends will see it as such. Those I hold in confidence know what I'm talking about, some, more than others.

With all of that being said I'll say this now. Don't try to rub my face in things that I don't care to see or if I sidestep them, then I didn't want to talk about or see pictures of! Again, those closest to me know what I'm talking about and I'm certain those who are doing this may get the idea. Don't Force me to be cruel. Don't make me have to take my friendship elsewhere when I offered it earnestly and whole heatedly. I won't call you people out, but I have friends who will. I won't stir up things, but I have two sisters, maybe three, who will, to defend me from any more mental anguish. I'll leave this at this. Hopefully it'll be enough.

July 9, 2017

Ways to guarantee that you'll eventually get booted off my Facebook.

Drama: Maybe I may have been into it when I was younger, but I'm getting older now and my mental condition won't put up with it for long. Don't bring me your drama because I don't have any in my life! I remove all drama that comes to my life as quickly as possible! Can't take it, won't have it!

Endless whining: If you have to whine every single day about something on Facebook, that's closely akin to the drama thing. Yes, you may have things going wrong in your life. Yes, you may hurt every day of your life. Yes, there may be things wrong that you need prayer for. But life isn't about the bad things ALL the time! Everybody (including me) has things going wrong, and yes, every day! I'm not trying to be mean, believe me! If you can't find a thing in your life to praise God for, then you don't need to be in mine! Yes, I pray for everybody who needs it, EVERY day! It would be nice, however, to hear a praise report when those prayers that everyone is giving for you are

ANSWERED! And I know they are! Fact is, there's not a day in my life that I don't hurt, there isn't a day that I don't battle with depression and bipolar disorder, and there sure isn't a day that I don't worry, but I don't post it every single day. Let God handle some of it! He can, and He will!

Everybody hates me because: OMG, I hate this one the most! And I see it the most these days! I'm bisexual so everybody hates me. I'm gay so everybody hates me. I'm black so everybody hates me. I'm a transsexual so everybody hates me. I'm mixed so everybody hates me (I even hate myself). Blah, blah blah. That's such a crock! We all have something about us that is different! So everybody hates everybody else? I think not! And God forbid if I call one of my black friends black! Come on! You can call me white, but I can't call you black? Get off it! I'm basically heterosexual. They CALL me white, but I'm not. I'm female, but I don't ACT like many women. I'm not whimpering about any of my eclecticisms! Not a single one! We are diverse! All of us! And everybody is a generalization that we all need to learn to quit using! It's insulting to those of us who have a liberal enough mind that we accept other as they are; be it black, white, mixed, native American, gay, straight, bi, or metrosexual! And that's just a fact! Wanna get off my friends list? Keep it up! You'll see how fast I'll delete you because I don't condone it.

Everything has to do with politics: Dear Lord and baby Jesus, please take me away from this one! If I see too many more posts blaming Trump for this and Obama for that and this one for this and this one for that, I'm going to scream and just start going into my little box out back alone! When did the President of the US have omnipotent domain? I didn't know we had a King or Queen of the USA. I thought we had a Senate and House of Representatives that were helping to screw things up! I thought we learned all this in 5th grade! But someone obviously wasn't paying attention. A lot of you weren't paying attention. If you're so stupid that you think ONE man or woman can make ALL the decisions and mess things up for EVERYBODY in a certain class, you desperately need help. But I'm NOT going to argue with you over it. I'm not going to stress myself out over it. I'll just delete you and go on with my life.

Pet peeve and real way to get kicked: Hit on me. I'm not talking about asking to go out and have a good time or see each other as friends. That isn't what I'm talking about at all. I'm talking about guys who hit on me thinking I'm hard up for a man, so they can just talk to me any way at all. Or they're married (and I won't call anybody out, but you know who you are) and they're wanting to cheat on their wife, so they want to see me (like I'm a slut or something because I'm not with somebody). Now the ones who let it drop after they asked, I've let go. The ones who won't shut up, like I have to have a man to be fulfilled or something or I have to have sex to be happy, those are the ones I end up deleting. Or the ones that think because I'm single that I WANT to be married. Maybe (and this is just facts) I don't. Maybe I just as well not have that obligation again (which may or may not be true). And I get told that a woman needs a man. Who told you that lie? I don't. Through the last two marriages and one of the last three relationships after that, I didn't NEED a man. I taught my kids' father how to do brakes on a car, how to change oil on a car, how to change the gas filter, how to strip paint, how to tile floors, and how to do a lot of other things. I had to do all of the grass cutting in that marriage and in the last one. I had to start doing the grass cutting here because it NEVER was getting finished by the last live in. I learned NOT to rely on a man for ANYTHING. But, I know I can rely on my boys if I need them to come running and get things done when I ask them to. I just don't ask unless I have to have the help. Oh, and the younger guys who hit on me thinking they're going to get a free ride (both ways), forget it. I don't want or need that either. You might be pretty to look at, but I'm not raising any more kids. I've got two of my own and that's enough. I've taken a total of 4 men from being inadequate to being efficient and been crapped on, so no thanks. I'm learning what to look for quickly. Wanna get deleted? Push me. Wanna be my friend and be with me? Let me take my time. Don't push. And let me be Angie.

I know there's more that I was going to say, but I think this may have gotten me into the stink with about half my friends' list anyway. I'm going to leave this here. Trust me, I don't hate a soul. But I love me more than I love you. I have to. I have a family to take care of. And I'm going to live to be 100

.

October 13, 2017

Welcome to another episode of the Stomach Turns, starring ME! Just for shits and giggles friends and neighbors, here's a recap: When we last left our heroine she was knee deep in debt, wondering where she'd find a job again, and thinking she may have found a man she could spend her golden years with.

Well, somebody PLEASE hit the magic buzzer, because Nope! At least one of those things ain't happening.

I'm still in debt and probably always will be – no big thing there. I have a job that I actually like that doesn't wear me out and doesn't suck.

Oh and the last thing? Well, the guy could have been THE ONE. He should have been. But – damn alcohol – I can't deal with a heavy drinker/alcoholic again. (And she pulls her drawing board back into the room)

I honestly am at the point where I either give up and just be me or I get really depressed. After all, we've seen that I'm not a not a good wife/girlfriend, right? I'm too independent now for my own good. Having nine years of the cheater and four years before that with a man who was afraid to love me made me strong, independent and hard, I guess.

Life experiences outside of relationships have made me distrustful even more. And as far as love goes, the last man I THOUGHT I love wanted to control and use me. And thank God I woke up before he got his hooks into my money, home, and property like he was trying to.

If I'm only good for someone to use; if I'm just a stepping stone in the pond of life, then I guess from now on, everyone who's on this path is gonna drown. This stepping stone just stopped being there. Either she moved or sank: Your pick.

For this Friday the 13th edition of our story, I'll be adding more to show exactly who I am.

I think it's time everyone saw me for the monster I really am, so this journal entry will actually enlighten you. I'm tired of caring what people think of me. Either you like me, you love me, or you don't. I'm not making up to you or begging you to care for me or be my friend. Personally, I think I'm pretty damned terrific. If you don't agree, I'm sorry for you. But I'm not going to apologize anymore for being me.

I'm smart, funny, and I love life with a passion that very few have ever known. And when I love you, I love you all the way. I see your faults but I love you regardless of them. You don't find that often anymore.

And what of me? Well, I'll live because I will live. I'll live because God and I have made an understanding. I'll live, happy or sad. I'll live because I must! I may get old and die alone, but I will NEVER compromise who I am for another person. I have to be myself. To paraphrase Harley Quinn: I go "where I want, when I want, with who I want." And that's just how it is. I feel lonely sometime. I wish I was more like other people but I know I'm not and I never will be.

I have ups and downs like a rollercoaster on some days. I can't make myself take a medication that's going to make me feel odd, have an allergic reaction, or that may kill me in the long run. I would rather deal with it. And the things in my head make me different. They make me not fit in. They, at times, make me a monster. In the same light, they also make me funny and sensitive. They make me charming.

Let's face it, I'm a walking contradiction. No wonder no one can really love me.

(And she laughed out loud at her own revelation.)

Another reason I don't have a man: It can be summed up, I guess, by one of my BFFs the last time he saw me. He just said it point blank and to the point. "What happened to you, Angie? You used to fix your hair and do up a little bit." What he didn't know and is about to find out with the rest of the world is that make up isn't me. I do try to get my hair decent, but your decent may not be mine.

Fact: If a guy can't deal with a woman who's about as unfake as they come, they're not gonna want to be with me. Anyway, they meet me sometimes and see me for who I am – a MONSTER. And they're done. Or, like two guys in the past few years, they thought since I was alone, I was hard up enough I'd beg for their attention. Sorry, boys, I may not be beautiful, but I'm sure secure enough that I'll NEVER beg for anyone's affections. And I'll never be used for mine again, either. Or my money (like, oh yeah, I'm rich!) or my home (like, I'm the queen of my double wide mansion!). The whole bowl of gumbo is right here: This old girl ain't hard up. I might not be the prettiest flower in the meadow, but damned if I won't grow the strongest and bloom the longest!

Having only one hour of sleep will make for a very prolific day. It will also make you remember that you had two male friends who have thought enough of you that though they love you and advances were made on both parts, the respect was there. You didn't get used because they valued the friendship too much. And almost identical words were spoken. "I don't want to lose you, Angie. You mean too much to me to let something physical come between us." Those words mean more to me than all the other men and their pretty words, their petty, "I love yous" or "I'm falling for you" or any other number of lies I've been told.

My heart aches when I reminisce and hear my own children's father saying, "I don't know if I love you or if you're just good in bed." Every so often, even after all these years, I hear it. It makes my teeth (what few I have left) gnash and my skin crawl. I want to cry and scream and beat up grass. It makes me want to take my sledgehammer to his grave and just pound the dirt or anything else I can hit. But he wasn't the only one who ever said anything similar. I can't beat them all. All I can do is say, man, I've had a messed up life.

October 20, 2017

My mind was prattling this off this morning, shortly after my eyes opened. I'm not entirely sure I wasn't thinking about it in my sleep. Fact remains that it is an absolute fact. And an absolute truth as well.

I am an addict. The seeds of addiction were sown young in me, planted deep and watered regularly with good intentions that ended up doing much more damage than good.

With the addiction card having been played, let me explain what addiction really is, in fact: Addiction is a driving desire for anything in or to excess. It is a compulsion, whether acted upon or not, that drives an individual in some way. And whether or not that person will admit it, it is there.

So, when I say I'm an addict, oh yes, I'm very serious.

And addicted to more than one thing, as well.

My first addiction started at a young age. For what it's worth, it's something we all would die without. That's right, you guessed it: Food.

Now please don't get me wrong, I'm not blaming a soul for the way I've continued to eat my feelings over the years. For the better part of my life, I've spent it destroying my body with yo-yo weight loss and gain, fad diets, starvation diets, nd anything I could, to attempt to make this body into something that a man (and myself) would want to look at for more than five seconds without becoming nauseated.

Just the facts, Jack.

It's unfortunate that once I've worked and worked to near exhaustion to do this (always failing miserably) that I revert to the addiction. And I eat to cover the feelings of failure and rejection. Usually I end up at least 5 to 10 pounds heavier than I was when I started. And I always get the same old blather from people: "You have such a beautiful heart (soul)."

No one looks at that. And the fat makes me slow and clumsier than I already am. If the heart really mattered so much, why am I alone? As I sit here writing this, I find myself wishing for a huge plate of nachos, so I could just munch the pain away. Because besides destroying my health over the years with the yo-yos, I've also managed to get my self esteem flattened quite a bit, too.

Addiction #2

This one won't be shared on social media and if asked, I'll totally refuse to comment because it's nothing I'm proud of.

I was and still am addicted to sex. I hate it, but I love it. And it's so horrible that my morals are ripping the part of me that has been around the block more than a few times to shreds now. Even as I was enjoying myself, a part of me was screaming that it was wrong, and I shouldn't be doing this. But the part of me that is so addicted to the gut wrenching, sheet ripping, back clawing pleasure of orgasm did not care.

With menopause came painful sex, but after the first few moments of searing pain, the pleasure took over. My drive was and is only dampened by the memories of the pain, the horrible treatment I received from my live-in, and my own self loathing for not standing up to him and tossing him out on his head for mistreating me.

He wasn't that good in bed. He just was there. So, for nine years, I tolerated it because it was regular sex, if nothing else.

Oh my God, I sound horrible. I loved his kids. I still do. But as for loving him, I think that died after the first six months.

I honestly didn't want to lose his friendship. For a while.

Then, I didn't even care about that anymore, because it just didn't matter. I had pushed myself into his mold for so long, I'm not sure I'll ever be me again. And all for the sake of a little (less than subpar, actually) regular sex.

Dear Lord, forgive me.

I honestly think had I not been cheated on, verbally abused, and raped while I was in this last relationship, my entire outlook would have been a lot different.

But such is life. And I must go on.

Addiction #3

Nicotine-Oh joy, oh joy!

Whoever made cigarettes should've been shot on sight.

After fighting the nicotine dragon for almost 50 years, I've tried everything from patches to hypnosis to quit smoking. Nothing has worked for long. Sadly, I don't think anything will.

Turkey Buzzard *Angela Luck*

Hilariously, I even named my dog in honor of smoking, because I am painfully aware that I'll probably die before I quit this habit. Maybe something will click in my head one day that will allow me to quit without gaining a huge bunch of weight. I'm finally under 200 pounds and I would love to stay that way.

I don't want to pick back up one addiction for another.

Oh, and by the way, my dog's registered name is Luck's Champion Smoke 'Em if Ya Got 'Em, Sig, for short. And yes, he's a full-blooded Australian Shepherd Mini.

At any rate, enough about addictions. There are more, trust me. But I think I've said enough. For now.

Every part of my life is screwed up in some way by my addictions.

Turkey Buzzard   Angela Luck

October 29, 2017

I'm seriously at the point I don't care anymore. I slept with someone who I've known for a few years online, but didn't have a good working personal relationship with, just because he was physically attractive to me. And I don't care anymore.

I think it had to have been a mistake because I'm sure he has taken me for a loose woman. Honestly, my heart has been hurt so many times now, I think I've just shut most of it down. It's not funny anymore. It's best for me just to turn my heart off. Just give up on finding someone who will just want to enjoy my company. I guess being me and being good in bed (yes, I guess I am) makes having a heart a liability.

It also makes wanting to serve God a liability sometimes (but only to myself). I only want one man at a time but I'm not sure I didn't make myself into a booty call for him. I'm just praying I didn't fuck it up.

It's not like I'm vested, but rather, because I feel guilty over it. I taught my sons one thing and I do another. So not right.

Turkey Buzzard   *Angela Luck*
November 3, 2017

Makes you want to start out, like, "Dear Diary", or something, right? But this isn't really a diary. It's my ramblings that I'm using in an attempt to keep sane. Not working real well right now, either.

I don't want to go nuts and lose the best job I've ever had because I crash and burn.

This is so hard. Every day it gets harder and harder to keep it together. I need help.

If my copay on therapy wasn't so much, I'd go, but it's just too much when 45 bucks can buy so many other things. Like boots or sneaks or food. Shirts to replace the ones I've ruined. Bedding. A carport. All kinds of things. Half of getting a tooth pulled. Come on, December.

New glasses. Come on March.

Turkey Buzzard   *Angela Luck*

November 5, 2017

Well, here goes. Another chapter of Days of Our MEH!

Today I write so I can get this off my chest. And it ain't my boobs! But it's about a boob, I'll guess. We'll see.

Not naming names. I try not to unless I'm just really fed up. And I'm not. I'm disappointed. But that ain't nothing but a thang. I'm gonna write in dialect sometimes the same as I say it, because he's not got the guts, I suppose to talk to me.

Thank God I'm not like I was when I was a kid. I don't get vested in people quickly anymore. That's a fact. I'm glad now that I don't, because you don't have the guts to tell me you're not interested anymore.

Fine by me. I wasn't really looking when you found me, and I'll be just fine as I am right now, without you. I've always got something to do with my life.

I found karaoke again. I suck at it, which is where I started 30 years ago. No biggie there. It makes me feel free. And I don't need you for that.

Once I found out your nature (purely by mistake), I found I would always just be a booty call anyway. No biggie in that either. After all, we all make mistakes

Turkey Buzzard *Angela Luck*

and boy, did I ever make one. All I can say is it ain't my first and I'll lay you a dollar to a donut it won't be my last.

Since you don't mean a thing to me besides a possible friendship that I totally screwed the pooch on, I'm not all torn up and it ain't like I'll go all chains and shotguns if I see you with someone else. I won't.

Ask a few of my men friends. They'll tell ya.

As long as we part on good terms, we're gravy.

Some, we didn't part on good terms to begin with, but we found our gravy later. Don't break it to where it can't be fixed.

Lies are what break a relationship, including a friendship. Be honest. That's just the truth.

November 11, 2017

Here is my luck with men:

The one I trusted locally did me wrong and actually thinks I'm too stupid to know it. The only one I totally know is trustworthy and would never do me wrong or cheat or lie and is actually adult enough to be a real man as well as a friend lives an hour from me. Oh, and if that isn't enough, my ultra-long-distance love and longtime friend has me considering moving again after my house is paid off. (Like that's gonna happen). But there are days I just want to run away.

There are days I wish seriously that I could pack my hedonistic retrosexual ass into a box and mail myself to Tahiti or Abu Dhabi or (God forbid) Colorado. Anywhere but here. Anytime but this century, sometimes.

I'm just so tired of loneliness and never finding anyone I can trust. If I give in, I'm a slut and if I hold back, I'm a tease. Where is the middle ground? Or if there any?

Turkey Buzzard   *Angela Luck*

I appear so calm. I smile. I act like I have it all under control.

Truth? The me that lives inside wants to run screaming into the night, terrifying the neighborhood. The me that lives inside wants to run headlong into a brick wall just to see how much it'll hurt, because no physical pain could cap the mental agony that it is to be me. The me that no one sees wants to know what it feels like to be hit by a car because maybe, just maybe, the escalation and flying into the air will help me escape this prison of hopelessness I live in every day.

See? Being used, being lied to, having your heart ripped from your chest way too many times creates a very damaged individual. And that individual is me.

And why don't try to kill myself? Because as black and as bleak as life is, it is far better than the pit of darkness and uncertainty that is death for me right now. It's not like I don't believe because I do. God heals, he gives life, he gives hope for life beyond death, and he also punishes. I'm not so sure that if I died, there wouldn't be even more punishment on the other side waiting for me, before I even get a glimpse of heaven. You see, I've not always been a sweet little innocent person. I've done a lot of wrong. My belief is that not all wrong can be repented and forgiven. You've got to pay for some of it. I'm paying now and who's to say, besides God, when I've paid enough? And since no man may know the mind of God, then I don't know it either.

There will be a lot who will tell me how wrong I am. That's fine. You are all entitled to disagree with me. I don't pick my friends based on their religious beliefs, & I hope most of you don't. I would like for you to know I believe in miracles and I know God works them every day. I don't look for one for myself, but I know I will get back my semblance of happiness in a few days to a week or a month. My life and point of view never depended on being attached anyway. I just am very badly missing karaoke and my friends. It makes me reflect on everything, but I shall survive!

For those who lasted through this latest rant, thank you for reading my words. I do mean it when I say I love you all.

Turkey Buzzard   *Angela Luck*

Bright blessings and may God be with you.

November 12, 2017

Something always screws things up for me.

Ok

Whatever.

I refuse to quit. I refuse to give up and lay down and say that's it. It's never the end for me. It never will be.

I'll leave this world with music in my heart and my toes tapping to the rhythm as a hold one of my family's hands and smile at them.

I hope I remember to tell them, "I wouldn't change a thing about this life. It's been a helluva ride!"

I have lived just like I'll die. Loving my kids and family and doing all I could for them. Trying to be as selfless and hopeful as I could and laughing in the face of heartache, danger, and fear. Showing my kids and the world that I may get down, but I'm never out.

Teaching those who will simply listen that we are all human and everyone should be treated with respect regardless of age, sex, race, religion, or sexual orientation. Oh, and let's add one more to the group—no, two—size and appearance.

Turkey Buzzard   *Angela Luck*

I'm back in my element today, even
though I'm sort of lamenting my inability
to sing like I used to. It's all good. So, I
won't go to AGT. Big deal.

November 14, 2017

Sometimes I just want to ask one certain friend and he knows who he is why I wasn't good enough to be anything but a FWB, and his excuse was he'd never have another girlfriend but now he's got one. He had the nerve to criticize me but turned his back on me when I turned down the FWB offer because that's not what I'm about.

Some days it just doesn't pay me to think because I end up putting myself down again.

I'm not ugly. A very handsome man came by my work today just to see me and give me a kiss, so I know I'm not ugly. And I don't need all that make-up and hair spray and crap. I don't have time for it. God gave me curls and he's blessed me. I've finally learned what to do with them, too.

I'm not dumb either. I'm probably one of the smartest people I know. I've got almost ten years of college, maintained a 3.8 GPA into my fifties, managed to get one degree and almost two more and my CNA 2. I'm a published author and I'm writing more now to publish in the future. Although I'm not perfect in my line of work, I love it and the people I encounter.

Turkey Buzzard   Angela Luck

Sometimes I just get angry at being treated like I'm second class, though, by someone I thought was a friend. I hope he reads this and knows my feelings have been badly hurt, not so much by the fact that he wouldn't date me (because I probably wouldn't have said yes if he'd asked), but because of the way he was supposed to have been my friend and treated me like I was less than a piece of trash, how he took credit for my hard work at getting some things going, and how he knows because I have more integrity than he'll ever have, I'll never call him out by name on it. I don't begrudge his happiness, but I sure feel kicked as a friend and I can assure you all, I won't be there next time he needs my help.

I'd like to thank my darling folks who have stood by me and still build me up. I know I'm not perfect and I know I'm not everyone's cup of tea either. I'm just glad someone cares. I think I've ranted enough for one night. Thanks again.

Turkey Buzzard *Angela Luck*

Turkey Buzzard   *Angela Luck*

November 15, 2017

The mirror tells me more than pictures. I have wrinkles and scars. I'm getting old. Do I accept it or fight it? I can fight what age is trying to do to my body and I can win but the ravages of time in my face, I can't. I refuse to pile makeup on in any attempt to hide who I really am. And if my looks are all that matters, fuck everything.

I'm so tired of this. Tired of being alone. Tired of being not good enough. Tired of being used. If it wasn't for my kids and my animals I swear I'd give up and just go back in my hole to stay. One won't let me come to his house. One won't come out to meet me. One is too busy. One's way too far away. And my meds are the only reason I'm not crying tears that need to flow.

I need to feel something outside. But I don't.

All I feel is that emotion of mine pouring through the hole in my heart that Hutchins left behind, and Stinnett made bigger when he dropped me for asking him to slow down and was engaged within a month. Anything that anyone else has done that should have hurt me or should have made me cry just floats through that huge hole, founders around a while, and drifts back out with the tide.

I try to be nice, instead of the bitch I know I can be. I wasn't raised to act the way men want me to! Is there anything wrong with being strong, intelligent, honest and forthright? Is there anything wrong with wanting a real date? Dammit, why did Coty have to die? He, honestly, was, the last true gentleman. He wanted to be a man. To take me out and he wasn't ever ashamed of me, no matter what I did. Only one other ever treated me that way that I remember. And he's still my friend to this day. His family welcomed me and mine like him. But I guess maybe the miles between us kept us apart. I don't want to guess anymore because that was a lot of years ago. It makes me want to be sad and it just flows through my heart again.

November 25, 2017

No one in my life for keeps. I'm not happy about it, but I'm not actively looking either.

I think if the last two men I was with felt that they had to bypass me to marry someone else, maybe there is something wrong with me. And if you really want to get technical, it's more like the last 5 men I've dated moved on to marry someone else.

The more I think about it, the sicker I get.

I feel like there's never been a man who truly loved me in my entire life. Not romantically. Maybe it's better that it just stops now. Maybe it's time for me to give up and just let myself go. Be mother to my kids. Try to get to see my daughter and my grandkids (not blood daughter, but at the time I originally wrote this, I felt like she really was my daughter. I learned she didn't feel the same, later).

I know I need to face it that I'm not, never was, and never will be a pretty woman. If I wore make up, I'd appear a lot prettier, but I just can't find time, nor can I see to do my eyes anymore. I always felt that over half of make up was the eyes. So, I just gave up. I have very few teeth left, and I see people (even those who are supposed to be my friends) laughing at me behind their hands or whispering about me in each other's ears. I learned to read lips at Wix, years ago. It's not that hard and I know what I saw.

I got moved off the front line at Love's, not because I was slow, but because of my looks. I know tis for a fact. And I was fired for the same reason (if they can't make you quit, they make up something that isn't true and get several people to lie and say it is). Just to think: I cried over losing that job.

I'm afraid to meet new people because I know I get judged on my looks. Guys don't want to take a woman out who looks like me. Just truth. Oh, I'm fine until I open my mouth.

Yeah, I'm good enough to see in private, but they're ashamed for their friends to see them with me. In other words, I'm good enough to have sex with, but not good enough for their friends or family. Now all of this is hypothetical, because the people who know me know that I don't go around screwing every man I date, talk to, or invite to my house.

And please, don't say, go get dentures or whatever. I have things that are more important than dentures. My self-esteem

Turkey Buzzard   *Angela Luck*

and confidence aren't, hasn't, and will never be at the top of my list. I have a home with a heat pump that's not working. My windows are all melted shut.

So much needs to be done.

I seriously don't know which way to turn.

Turkey Buzzard — Angela Luck

December 3, 2017

Unbelievable. Just unbelievable.

I seriously don't know what is more shocking to me: The fact that it's December of 2017 already or the fact that I've managed to blow up three or four crappy would-be relationships and maybe two or three possible good ones.

Not that I give a rat's ass anymore. I take medication to keep me from showing that I care.

I had an insurance salesman tell me yesterday that we weren't meant to be alone. I wanted to laugh in his face. I know it wasn't the way God intended it. God created man and woman to be together as companions, help mates, friends. But for the original sin, committed by a woman, I sure have taken a lot of lumps from men in my day and just lately, too.

I just keep asking myself, "Why do I keep doing this?" "Why don't I just give up?" The day I give up is getting closer and closer.

One more heartache. And I honestly keep praying this heartache will be the one that kills the last bit of hope, the last glimmer of that shiny silver lining I keep seeing, praying my heart finally turns

Turkey Buzzard — Angela Luck

totally black, so I can hurt no more. It never happens, but I pray for it.

So, when you see me and see no mirth in my cold blue eyes, just know that a world of heartless people who have kept twisting the knife of rejection and pain have helped to make this soul what it is today. When you see me smile and it doesn't seem quite right anymore, know I've had to paint on grins to mask everything from abuse to anger to even rape, (which, no, I will not go into and don't ask).

Know that when and if I am truly happy (on rare occasions), I'm still having a very hard time showing it. My self-consciousness about my appearance is only compounded by loosing my teeth, constantly fluctuation weight, wrinkles, and scars that will never go away.

A real smile is a nightmare for me. And when somebody who has, themselves, been hit by the ravages of age, says, "If you turn me on, we'll go from there," I'm sorry, but I'm not in this to turn you on.

I dress for me. I do my hair for me. I act like me. If I run men off, oh well. If I make women mad, too bad. And even though I don't show my feelings, I still have them, so don't make fun of me or laugh behind my back. That hurts more than saying it to my face. Have the guts to say your mind to me!

I guess I've just cared about the wrong people. That's why I'm just seriously thinking of giving up.

Maybe if I pray hard enough, God will help me just turn everything off. I need to focus on my family and close friends. Just kill every other emotion. I need to stop feeling like I'm not good enough.

I need to stop being sentimental and sending someone a song that obviously means nothing to them. It doesn't matter to them that it struck a chord with me. I need to stop thinking that anyone is EVER going to change. Once a two-timer, always a two-timer. Once a dirty old man, always one. Stop trusting someone who hasn't given me a reason to trust them.

God provided the way to get the windows and heat pump fixed. I need to put my faith in him to help me not to be lonely anymore. I need to ask God to help me close the hole that's in my heart bigger than ever because of yet another man making me feel like I'm nothing.

I'm sitting here at work, fighting tears that I don't even know why I want to cry. All I do know, is that this has to stop. If someone can't be with me or friends with me for the right reasons, I don't need them at all. When it makes me feel this way, something is so wrong. I think its time I stopped. Before I get myself too far gone.

THUS SAITH THE MAJICK

December 8, 2017

Today, revelations without libations, as usual. Writing affected makes for some pretty poor writing sometimes. Other, perhaps, fairly gifted, but I've found that words brought on by an overindulgence in any substance could be referred to as intellectual drivel at best. My experience, no one else's.

In defense of the inebriated, otherwise intoxicated authors of our time and the past, I applaud you. You have given the world works of art that shall never be repeated, of that I am sure. I, personally, prefer and am able to create much more clearly with a bottle of water and a pack of M&Ms. Of course, I'm lining the M&Ms up in like colors, choosing my favorite color for last because for some ungodly reason it just tastes better that way.

Then, deciding what could the odd ones would make if you chewed the candy shells together in your mouth all at once and doing it because suddenly, I don't really want to think about it.

There are actually days I think of my life as a dream. And not a bad one. More like a fairy tale. Evil has been beaten, curses broke, villains conquered and the wicked vanquished before there can be a happy ending.

Once you realize that stories told of evil queens, dragons, witches, and all sorts of trials to overcome, you see that a fairytale isn't all it's cracked up to be in the first place. We all live a fairytale existence or can, if our response is right. It's all in how you treat oppression, obstacles, disasters, sadness, loss, and, yes, even death. So wherein lies the key to living a dream instead of a nightmare? How do you turn a struggle against what appears to be in surmountable odds into an opportunity? It's all about attitude, my friends. And, for the most part, I have to say I have a winning one. I may not feel that I belong in a relationship or that I even can keep one going or deserving of one, but at life I AM a winner.

Now there will be (as there always are) a faction of people who will say or comment "How can you say that? You're not set in life. You're not well off. You live in a trailer! You're disabled, and you work part-time in a gas station!"

Being a winner has nothing to do with status as fat as money, job, even social standing. Being a winner is defined in how you handle what you have encountered in your life. It also has to do with admission of your own shortcomings and willingness to do what makes you happy and not necessarily what makes the most money. Winning has to do with not only making yourself happy but delighting those you encounter and filling the occupation you were designed for by God.

Part 2

Confusion. One thing that eats my soul. I know beyond a shadow of a doubt that there are people who, if I state a few things, can and will be hurt or made angry by my words or actions. I seriously and honestly don't want to harm a soul.

Therein lies the confusion.

What do I do?

December 21, 2017

I swear, every man I meet only wants sex. Pigs! Just plain pigs!

Not one is looking for a friend or companion first. No one wants to give true love a chance. Glen was the king of all pigs! He was so nice on the phone, then once we met all he wanted to do was meet up somewhere and have sex in the car! I'm not a teenager and I'm sure not a whore!

I have a younger man friend who would love to go out, but again, it switches to sex after we've talked a while. And I'm not sure I'll ever want to see a younger man again.

I'm not sure I want a man at all anymore. I just want someone who will love me. I'm about to switch sexes. I swear. If I really thought I could this late in the game, I would.

I can see from my own writing, just how much my mental illness is playing with my entire being. At least, knowing helps me. I know I'm sick and I have to be careful. I could end up doing some really dumb shit.

December 31, 2017

This year is over. And ending it on a positive note here. I've got a very good job, a warm home, wonderful family, good health for the most part, a good man friend in my life, and I'm so blessed by God.

2017 hasn't been without its trials and tribulations. But this is something we all must face in life. Fighting to continue is worth all the gain received in the end. Faith is the earth, hope, the water, and love, the fertilizer, for blessings abounding. Everything happens for a reason and with faith and belief that the Lord will reveal that reason, good things can and will spring forth.

Resolutions? Not a one. Things I'd like for 2018? Happy life (got it). Continued friendships. Better health (working on it). More ways to serve God. To be able to write more on my books.

Turkey Buzzard　　　　　　　　*Angela Luck*

As this world gets more and more evil, we should cling to those who matter to us tighter and tighter

Sometimes you're too busy protecting others From The Storm to realize that you've been struck by lightning.

Things that help bipolar and other personality disorders.

There are just plain facts and that is all. Granted, disorders that are considered or have been found to be caused by chemical imbalance in the brain still require proper medical treatment, as well as a few other things that the patient or their family can do to help stabilize the affected person. Having this disease and realizing that I was one of the ones strongly affected by it, has led me to try to assist others, so they can perhaps enjoy the more normal life I never had until I was much older. I'm not even saying I'm at 100%, because I'm not and I never will be. However, some things do help with stability.

1. Established routine: Even if you have to set reminders on your phone or get someone else to nudge you, start getting into some type of routine. Go to bed and get up at a certain time every day. Eat your meals at a certain time. Do things according to schedule.
2. Balance your diet. I'm as guilty as every other person who has a personality disorder on this one. Binge diets. Then diets to lose. Starvation. That isn't a way to lose weight or to keep your

disorder in check, either. A good balanced diet, with 2 small snacks a day, is essential to not only a healthy body but a healthier mind. Don't believe me? Try it for a month and see.

3. Get out in the fresh air and sunshine. Not saying you have to have a stringent exercise routine. Just get outside and walk. Enjoy the sun! Breathe in life! It's a fact that people who enjoy at least 30 minutes of activity every day tend to live longer and have a better outlook. Further, those with a better outlook on life and who embrace life are 75-85% less likely to commit suicide. These are my figures, but I'm pretty close to being right, if not dead on.

I'm always writing things that I think may help others. I hope this will help someone somewhere.

January 5, 2018

"Not everyone can live in a fairy tale or has a fairy tale life (love)." Well, thank God! I don't want a fairytale, myself! Fairytale love is bullshit. It's not real.

Let me explain something to you. And this is reality, truth, fact, or whatever you want to see *real life* as. There is no happily ever after because people die. Hence there is **NO Fairytale**.

Further, anyone who has half a brain know that there's always strife, a witch or two, or a poison apple in a fairytale, right? So, what's so perfect about it? Not a thing!

Why rant? Seriously, no reason. Just hit me suddenly that I'd never really replied to Stinnett's la-de-da bullshit trying to get me to break down. His comment of, "I guess I expected too much after 28 years in a fairytale" left me so aghast at the time, I had no answer. In afterthought, it sounds more like 28 years mostly of laying in bed to me.

From my experience, it was laying in bed groping each other and ignoring their kids. No wonder they were all heathens. And if he still has custody of his grands, they're fixing to be the same way.

Turkey Buzzard   *Angela Luck*

And you wonder why I didn't want your "fairytale"? Yeah, right.

You sell over half of your meds every month to make ends meet, allow your adult kid to smoke weed in the house around a six-year-old who has ADHD, then proceed to throw the same six-year-old out of your room when he wants attention, but you want "private time"? Yes, I know all this for a fact. How's that fairytale, now?

I think I'll just keep mine, thank you. At least I know that if the relationship part doesn't work out, we'll stay friends as we've always done. I know all both of us want from each other is companionship, respect, and love. We're not after each other's money or property or anything else. Oh yeah, and if one of us doesn't get their way, we don't pout, pretend to be sick, act suicidal or stir up drama.

He makes me laugh every day. I hope I at least bring a smile to his face. I think I'm finished because I don't have to explain anything to anyone.

Honey, you know how I feel.

And yeah, maybe this is a fairytale after all.

Thus Saith the Majick

January 19, 2018

Seems like nobody cares about keeping the house clean but me. I'm about to just give up.

Seriously, seems like no one much cares about me except for me, right now.

I truly do love my guy, just not as passionately as with others. Time and pain have scarred us both. And it's hard to attempt something perfect when all that's ever been handed to you has been burnt to ashes every time you turned around.

Damaged souls tend to cleave together. I don't know why, but they do. In a perfect world, maybe this would be good and helpful and right. This world is so far from perfect. Others don't even know they've hurt each other.

A thought for today:

It's hard to attempt something perfect when all that's ever been handed to you has been burnt to ashes every time you turn around. I'm sure time and pain has scarred everyone, but some have been scarred much worse than others. Don't judge a person by the fact that they don't

Turkey Buzzard   *Angela Luck*

want or can't commit to a passionate relationship. For some, the pain is just

too deep; the holes are just too big in their hearts.

February 1, 2018

Quickly heading into the year of the dog. A lot of folks just assume that 2018 is the year as we westerners see it.

Chinese New Year is actually February 16. It's still the year of the Fire Rooster.

My year is next year. Year of the Pig or Boar. I can't wait. It should be a year when things go very well for me.

I found this one and decided to include it from quite a while ago. Mr. H and I were together, but I knew it wasn't long until we'd be apart again for the 3rd time.

August 3, 2013

Of course, I know he's going to be leaving again before too much longer. Am I worried about it? Certainly not.

Does the thought make me sad? Yes, very, but I can't afford to show it.

Will I ever give my heart to another as I have him? Probably not ever.

I can't afford to let me pain show. So, stronger nerve pills and occasional bouts with beers and a sip or two of moonshine. Once in a while, I go into my room, into my shower, and cry my eyes out. Those tears that I know I must occasionally allow myself, in order to keep from going out of my mind. That is the place that I dare not go.

Do I truly love him? The answer is an unequivocal yes. But through all the lies, all the cheating, and the leaving, I can't ever allow myself to trust him ever again enough to feel the pure love I had for him to begin with.

So, I hold my heart. I only fully love my family and myself. That includes my sisters and brothers whom I've adopted as mine along the way and 2 nieces, both of whom have no relation to me at all.

My life? It was happier when I was sure of things.

February 8, 2018

Thoughts:

I don't know what I want. I don't want to leave my guy hanging. I do love him to death but tasting the life and living it is two different things. The taste? Oh, it's fun. I'd be lying if I didn't say that. But—big but—it's not where I want to be fifteen years from now. It's not what I want to be limited to. I've just got so much more I'm interested in. Truth.

And why can't I just let go? Just forget what happened and who I was with from 2007 until 2016? Just blot him out of my mind and life like the piece of flotsam that he is?

February 8, 2018 11:35 am

Be who you are.

Don't make yourself into someone else's vision of who you should be.

True happiness is in you.

Not in what others perceive you to be.

February 9, 2018

I just can't fit in with the lifestyle. I'm not there without emotional turmoil.

I can't be an angel outside and devil inside. Can't afford to risk having someone see me where we've been going and say something that gets back to work. My job is more important than that. I do love my job. I work for a great company. To lose it over something that isn't even my personal choice in lifestyle is ludicrous. I loved seeing him get his swagger back and knowing I'd done part of it, but I just ain't into what he is.

Worst of all, I want to see him do good but I'm starting to wonder if it's in him.

I plan for the future and try to make it happen. He just wants to live for today.

So much mental strain.

February 11, 2018   6:54 am

Believe in yourself. Don't let others perceptions of your worth project within.

You know who and what you're worth. Show it. Prove it to yourself everyday because YOU are the only one you have to impress!

February 16, 2018

Age ravages the body. Bipolar, depression, ALZ, and other chemical/mental disorders ravage the mind. We fight to keep our youth. We deny the fact that we're aging.

When did it become wrong to get old? Age is something to bear pride in. Health is what we allow to decline then say old age has gotten to us. We need to care for our health; guard it like a beautiful crystal, so it is with us into our older years.

Younger folks have been calling me "old" for years. My heart isn't old, so it really hasn't bothered me that much.

There is no shame is being old. There is no shame in being yourself. There is no shame in being young at heart. Just don't allow others to define your image of yourself.

February 17-27, 2018

Well here goes:

Karma. You can say you don't believe in it. In one way or another, it does exist. Biblically, it's expressed as a warning that whatever you do shall be returned to you threefold. Wiccans call it the Rule of Three, I believe. In almost every religion, there is a "return for the evil" you do. There is also, in the same light, a return for good.

Even witchcraft warns of spelling those who are undeserving of evil, due to a sort of "blowback" effect. It also warns against spelling for gain for self, to assist those who are undeserving and to do harm to others. Basically, same reasoning.

With all the warnings going around from all these different sources, it would seem that people would treat each other better, wouldn't it? It would surely seem, with all of the media immersion of our age, with how tech-savvy our world has become, with how much varied culture is available to everyone, people would get the picture by now and stop all this evil.

Is it just human nature for us all to be vindictive to others without consideration for the consequences? Is it in all our natures to cheat on each other? Is it natural that some of us are treated as throw away for our entire loves, while others are considered better for theirs?

Is it natural that some of us are treated as throwaways for our entire lives, while others are considered better for theirs?

Are some people just destined by karma or some other force of nature or God to be used and thrown to the side for their entire lives?

Even in what is supposed to be the greatest country in the world, there is and always has been, a caste system. Before anyone starts going off their proverbial chain or jumping on their own little golden high horse or fairy snowflake unicorn, hold up a minute, because it's not what any of you whining ninnies think it is.

Our country has been split into groups of haves and have-nots since colonial times. This has NOTHING to do with race, sex, sexual orientation, or national origin. Very few people in our society treat all people there same, no matter who they are. So, while you bunch of blithering nincompoops are screaming racism, sexism, or God knows what else in this country, you're looking down your nose at those who have invisible disabilities (yes, you are--don't lie), those who don't make as much money as you (please don't even get me started), those who choose to do menial labor (yes, of course, you're better than they are. Bullshit!), elderly citizens who are struggling to maintain their Independence (they should go to a nursing facility, right? I don't think so!), and just about anybody who doesn't agree with you and your politics (I'm usually one of them. Put up your Dukes and let's tango!) There is just so much more I could add to that little list of prejudices.

Finally, the final chapter of the throwaways and other garbage my brain spits out in the middle of the day when nobody's looking:

And what exactly is wrong with calling people what they are? Did our entire world all of a sudden turn into a world of soft hearted, oh-my-God mushy, gushy babies? I was going to use another word and, on second thought, I think I will: Pussies. An entire generation and a half, maybe more, of PUSSIES! Whiny babies who can't deal with anything anymore.

Turkey Buzzard *Angela Luck*

Oh, whaaaaa-youre fat-boo hoo. So? I went through that my entire life and I didn't let it get me down. I don't need a safe place and I sure as hell didn't have one in Junior high school when seven girls ganged up on me every day for half the year, either. I got bullied by seven at a time. I got beaten up. I didn't need a safe place then and I don't now. Screw them. They got my curse. I stayed like I was: fat and ugly. They got that way. Oh yeah,& blind too.

And just for shits and giggles, no, I'm not white. I'm two races. I may be more than that. I'm gonna find out one day.

And I'm gonna finish this daily rant from 2/17/2018 like this:

Whoever you are; "Be excellent to each other."

----Bill S. Preston

February 20, 2018

I do not want to be alone.

But—I do not like how I feel right now. I feel cramped, crushed, lorded over, or subservial.

I am who I am. And I am magnificent. I am independent and strong. I am aggressive, and I go after what I want.

My problem is, after I go after it, sometimes it bites me in the ass.

The ability to love others because of their differences, rather than attempting to change them, is the greatest love of all.

Turkey Buzzard   *Angela Luck*

February 23, 2018

Hardly any sleep again. It's becoming my life again. Nerves keeping me from sleeping. I have to dope up and zonk to sleep.

Chase sleeping pills with beer. You do what you have to do.

My sleep gets less and less.

My hands wake me up in the middle of the night, throbbing.

Still, I carry on like nothing is wrong. I have to.

March 4, 2018

Pain is near unbearable, nerves are beginning to fray. I have pushed myself to work for a while that I've not felt like working. I've smiled when I haven't felt like smiling.

I've tried my hardest to be nice even when I've not felt like it. Honestly, I've kissed one persons' ass when I felt like telling him off for talking down to me.

Just because I choose to do a job doesn't me it's all I'm qualified to do. Don't talk to me like I'm stupid.

I've been to college. I have one degree, one certificate and 6 more years in 3 other majors. Just because I got bored with one and ran out of money for the last one doesn't make me less than anyone else.

Some days I just don't feel appreciated. I feel like management thinks I'm an old idiot instead of a very seasoned and educated person.

Turkey Buzzard   *Angela Luck*

April 8, 2018

Honey just listen to what I've got to say. I have been married four times. I never once looked at myself as a failure because my marriage didn't work. You shouldn't either. You do not allow your status, whether married or single, to Define Who You Are. You define Who You Are by Who You Are. Feed on yourself. Be a strong independent woman. Find confidence in being you. You will see from this, that you don't need a man to Define you. You don't need anyone to Define you. And once you have achieved that, your life will become so much better than you have ever dreamed it would be. I know! And I love you no matter what!

That goes for man or woman. You have to be confident in yourself before you can be with someone else and make it work, anyway. Needy people jump from relationship to relationship. Be confident. I am! God doesn't make junk!

April 21, 2018

A strong woman doesn't whine. I'm not whining. I've gotten to the point that I don't care anymore. Why should I wear myself out trying to make something work when no one else wants to? Why should I do all the leg work? Why should I provide everything to the relationship and get nothing in return? I'm tired of feeling used. I'm so tired of feeling like I'm only good for sex. I'm tired of feeling unpretty most of the time. And I'm done.

From now on, if someone wants me, for a while they need to put forth the effort. If they don't think I'm worth it, then oh well. I came into this world alone and I can sure go out the same way.

April 26, 2018

I am truly trying to put my thoughts together, so they make sense and are completely understood. I don't want anyone to think that I'm depressed, because I'm not.

I believe the better word would be disheartened. When someone has tried to meet up with someone that they consider important in their lives numerous times, over many years, and keep being put off by first one thing and then another, it is becoming painfully obvious to me that I don't matter to this person. Or at least I don't matter this person the way that I thought I did.

Again I'm recording this here as a record so that I will have it, but also so perhaps someone else can see that this type of treatment actually does hurt someone sometimes.

I was good enough to ask for money, but I'm not good enough to come see you. I was good enough to ask for help when you needed help. I'm not good enough to be around you now that you don't need help. When you needed a place to stay, I'm plenty good enough for you to be around. But when you're happy, and things are going your way, and your life is grand, you don't want to share that part with me.

Being a friend in any measure or fashion, be it as a good friend, confidant, or considered as a family member, you should feel that I am good enough to be around you no matter what. If that's not the case, then why am I your friend? The answer is simple. You're not really my friend at all. I've been a friend to you, but you've not been a friend to me.

Friends are supposed to be there in good times and in bad. And if they can help each other good. If all they can be is a shoulder, that's good too. Being a true friend means that you can laugh together, cry together, and want each other's company no matter what. As far as I can see, I'm not trying anymore. Not with a few of my so-called friends.

This does not concern the ones of you whom I have spent lots and lots of time with and who I enjoy on a regular basis. It only concerns the very few who only want my friendship or my company when they need something.

After a while, I give up. With David, it was almost 9 years of seeing him cheat off and on. With my dad, it was 10 years of trying to get him just to talk to me. Those are two examples and there have been more. And it's okay. Because for every one of those people who I'm trying to make a life with, who I tried to be happy with, who I wanted to find joy with, I have found much better people in my life now than they are. So it's okay.

God bless you on your undertakings. I am through. I will try no more. My heart has taken the final blow. May you have a happy life, as I will.

I wrote this after a woman who I'd been close to since she was 18 years old and had considered her as a daughter told me she had not even 5 minutes for me to get to see her baby, who I consider my grandchild.

She was going to be close to where I live and I was willing to make the drive and even go to where she was going to be meeting up with friends, and meet her in a parking lot for 5 lousy minutes, just to be able to see my third granddaughter for probably the only time I'd ever get to see her. I was hurt.

I wrote her off in my mind.

But you can't tell my heart that she's written off occasionally. It still hurts badly, and I'll never forget the fact that when she was in dire straits, I was good enough for her to call Mama, but now that things are going well for her, she's ashamed of me, obviously.

It hurts my heart. And although she still calls me Mama on Facebook, it doesn't mean a thing to me anymore. Why? Because if it can't be carried into real life, it doesn't exist. And she can't keep hurting me, because although I come off as strong, I'm not.

May 10, 2018

I never looked with my eyes. And I got told that I needed to look better, to do more when I was waiting on someone hand and foot, that I needed to "do up" more, and got overlooked because I didn't look as good as other women, so don't preach to me about good men. I also got told I wasn't good enough to be anything but a FWB by a few men who I thought I respected until they said that! You must give respect to get respect! I have only given respect to this point, don't push me into more. I've always been nothing but a good woman. I just refuse to be treated like less anymore!

I just got called resentful and shallow because I made a comment about most men acting like little boys on a friend's timeline. I don't resent a thing! But almost everything I said in the previous paragraph came out of his mouth at one time or another! I've been honestly looked over I don't know how many times because I'm not as pretty as other women! And it came straight out of his mouth that he only wanted me as a FWB! So, respect? No, I don't respect you at all! And you resent my comment? More like you resemble my comment!

At least I'm mature enough to see that I'm not as pretty as other women. That doesn't mean I'm going to wear a ton of make up or kiss your ass to be loved by you or any other person. And you will note, I said person, not MAN. I'm who I am. But if you've gotta cheat on me and lie to me or treat me like trash, be you male or female, I DO NOT NEED the likes of you telling me that I'm freaking shallow!!!!

Before you call the kettle black, maybe you need to look at your own actions. You've hurt me more than you'll ever know by the way you treated me, acting like my "friend" in front of people and talking to me like you did in messenger and on the phone. At least I have the grand Elegance not to call your name so that everyone who knows you knows what kind of dog you really were to me.

Thank you. That is all.

June 7, 2018

The ultimate slap in the face: "Ok, if you say so." Why? Plain and probably not so simple because it really ticks me off. If I told you something then I said so, correct? Isn't this questioning the veracity of what I just said? Or wrote?

I, as a rule, am a fairly honest person. Why should I feel the need to lie to a soul in my life? I have none. No one in my life merits or needs to be disrespected in that way. Further, I have no one that I'm not close enough with in my inner circle, that they can't handle the truth.

There are things and events I'll keep inside myself until the day I die. Those things I've managed to bury deep enough that I barely can remember the details or even the dates and times. Much of it now has been pushed so far back behind the veil, it is but a gathering of spirits in a cloud of mist. It happened. It happened to someone: But I don't recall who it happed to unless forced or, as now, when I'm writing the spirits begin to regain their embodiment. Some even reclaim their names and faces. And the nightmare in my mind that I thought I had locked away becomes real to me again, if only for a few moments.

Those few moments end as my beloved gatekeepers, clad in the armor of my grandfather, grandmother, and Uncle Ode slam the gates of the mental dungeon again. Their smiles and the memory of the warmth of their love pushes the secret demons I harbor inside back into the murky depths where they belong. Where only I know they are there and ever existed. Where no one will ever know about what happened in those times and about the secret shame harbored in my soul that will never completely die.

So much pain and so much shame. So much sadness and a life ruined more than likely because of me. I keep shoving it back.

What I did was deplorable in any man's books and it made no difference that I had been raped and brutalized by several men by the time it happened.

It was one mistake. That one mistake was mine. Then I was blackmailed into more mistakes. OH! My God! I am so sorry. I had no right. Of course, I know I've paid and paid for it repeatedly, including more rapes, one near rape, failed relationships over and over, and seeing men I've adored marry or live with other women. Not to mention the one who is my weakness and the one who left a huge hole in my heart.

And not to mention being cheated on and lied about when I was doing nothing wrong, being pushed into cheating so he could hear about it later (it got him hot, but it made me sick) and more horrid things I do not wish to discuss.

Now, transcribing this, as with writing it the first time, I have to struggle to put this back away again. I have to find a way to bury this in the depths of my mind again, so it won't drive me batty. I have to make myself forgive myself. And yes, I've tried to talk to him to apologize, because even though he blackmailed me later, I was the one who gave him the ammo.

Needless to say, I've not been an angel, ever. Once again, I have to put the demon back in his lair. I'll never forgive myself for allowing hypersexuality to take control over me, no matter what.

Turkey Buzzard — Angela Luck

June 8, 2018

And this is how I write sometimes! Check the last of this for an update!

You ever feel like Karma has decided to kick your ass with steel toed army boots? Two very different men in your life mean the world to you and you don't or can't be with either one? One is so close to you that you literally can finish each other's sentences, but there's one huge deal breaker for you both? The other, well, you can't figure him out because he either doesn't want more than a part-time girlfriend, or thinks you're a slut, or is ashamed to be with you and you just don't know what to do about it? Then you're getting bombarded by people wanting money again and it's getting to where you don't know what to do anymore? You're scared to ask for help and you're too proud to ask for help, because you don't want anyone to know you're weak?

Meanwhile, you're not sleeping again? You're running into private restrooms or places where nobody knows you for 3 to 5 minutes, just so you can cry? And you know, know, know that part of this is God's way of thumping your head for being a bad, bad girl 20 or so years ago, and against all advisement from your Bible, you still ask him why? Haven't you

Turkey Buzzard   *Angela Luck*

been punished enough? Isn't all the abusive marriages, being taken advantage of, being cheated on; isn't it enough? Isn't 5 bankruptcies enough? Isn't losing everything you own except your kids enough? When will it ever stop?

Wasn't karma's stopping point when you lost your kid's father to an untimely death? Or was it when you found out he been lying about why he wasn't coming to see your children after you divorced? Was it when you found that he thought going across two states to see your divorced best friend was more important than his own children? Or was it when the next two men you cherished were taken from you: the first, by making you feel that money was more important than you were and the second by constant cheating and lying until the relationship was so cheapened you could never trust him again? Is it any wonder you keep asking Karma; asking God; asking the angels, why? Even after you've been so beaten down that your good heart feels like a lump of ash from being burned so much, that you can only cry alone since you feel tears are sign of weakness, you still feel the boot in your ass and you wonder when it will ever end.

Majick

And ya know what? the only one who even thought to check and find out if I was ok was Timmy!!!! Now that shows who really read this and who really does care, don't it?

Turkey Buzzard   Angela Luck

June 22, 2018

Not a rant: Just an observation.

Or should I say, a dirty truth?

And here goes.

There are just too many women in this world who are not getting the child support they deserve or (in some cases) not getting any support at all, because they are being stabbed in the back by money grubbing, gold digging, low-life bitches, who are hiding men that they KNOW should be paying support.

To me, this is just a crying shame.

Any woman who encourages a man NOT to take responsibility for the child or children that he fathered, to me, is the lowest form of female pond scum alive.

I don't care what the mother of the children is all about. It's not for us to judge. If the woman has custody and is raising your kid, it's your obligation, by law, and (in my mind and humble opinion) by God's moral imperative, to pay for your fair share to help with expenses of putting that child on Earth.

Any woman who is so selfish that she has to hide a man away from his children and take support from them by doing so or supporting him in working under the table, doesn't deserve to be called a woman and she certainly doesn't deserve respect from other women either.

Not only do her actions show insecurity, but a total disregard for others.

In order for a man to totally disregard his progeny, it takes a selfish spirit and sociopathic need to only please oneself.

For all intents and purposes, for a woman to allow her significant other to usurp his parental responsibility to his own children, is the lowest form of treason. Further, to in any way coerce him into mistreating his children is just vile and evil in the worst way.

But only God knows, in a world of psychotic women, narcissistic men, children who were damaged by nightmare parents with multiple partners (all of whom had to be called Daddy or Mama or the beatings began), and so much more, is it any wonder that some people can kill off one spouse, move quickly to the next, force their children on that one, and take the new one from their own children?

So, who is to say who's to blame? Is it our system? The woman, who is both enabler and facilitator? Or the man, who is the prognosticator or sociopath? Is it possible, both are sociopaths, feeding off one another?

Turkey Buzzard   *Angela Luck*

As or society changes and evolves, can it be said that we're not moving forward at all? Are we actually creating a breed of human that has little or no feelings at all, except for themselves?

Are we creating psychopaths, sociopaths, narcissists, and God knows the range of undesirable humanoid creatures, hiding in our midst under the human façade?

Think about it.

July 8, 2018

I'm one person who doesn't get enough sleep. I take sleeping pills yes, I do. But now let's explore a little bit of the myth and Truth behind insomnia.

The myth or the Superstition behind lack of sleep varies. One myth states that something that you've done is bothering you and your mind won't let you rest. Another variation is the devil won't let you rest. My personal favorite is the Superstition or belief that the angels are keeping you awake because something isn't right in your life. Perhaps that actual myth or superstition is closer to being the truth than the other variations, simply based in fact, since many who are unable to sleep need much more in their lives and aren't happy with what they have going on. Their subconscious won't allow them to rest, so they don't have to face the facts of their true feelings.

Other reasons for insomnia can be physical. Anything from pain to mental state can contribute to an insomnulent state that can last for days or weeks. As the mind continues to function without sleep, cognitive areas in the brain begin to falter. Waking dreams or hallucinations are not uncommon. Irritability, extreme sadness or depression or even anger can be part of the consequences of insomnia or interrupted sleep patterns.

How much sleep does an individual need? Some will say very little and others will say more. Ideally the sleep requirements for most people are between six and eight hours a night or day. It's not something that we can learn, it is actually something that is in our DNA. Our bodies were not created to function on less sleep, and we cannot teach our bodies to function much less sleep than 6 hours a night. Some people can function for a short period of time on less, but that's few and far between.

How can you manage to get to sleep and stay asleep? That is something that's plagued everyone who has ever had problems sleeping. It varies with the individual. And also depends on your DNA, your mental status, your physical health, and your sense of tiredness and well-being. To tell you to relax and clear your mind and is not going to work with every person. And a sleeping pill is not always the answer.

Just wanted to toss out some facts. I hope I've enlightened this day.

July 13, 2018

Start but never finish: Guilty.

Strangely, it's one of those "I don't know why" situations because the ideas and thought are still there. They just never seem to come to fruition.

Sounds crazy. Doesn't mean nothing.

I am not a traveler anymore. I enjoy the freedom of cutting grass, planting flowers or felling a tree. I am not a traveler. I enjoy warm afternoons on my back deck or under my tree out front with a cold glass of water or a beer and some good music playing.

I enjoy the hearts of my friends and family, freely given. I enjoy and love every one of my pets' personalities, all so different and uniquely devoted to me and my family.

I have changed. Yes, I found me but me was someone else. Me is a mostly quiet person with a pirate smile who wants her children to have a beautiful home after she's dead and gone and who would do anything to insure it for them.

Me became a dancer when she could not sing anymore. She became a fighter when she found that love didn't work anymore. She became a cynic when so many lied.

Turkey Buzzard   Angela Luck

She became ruthless when her heart was damaged so badly she wished she had died.

But through all of this, she became something else entirely.

To me, I became improved, better. More blessed and more alive. By closing doors to keep from harm's clutches, to protect myself and my loved ones from evil, I became a better version of myself.

I dance to all music of life. My heart, though oblivious to heartbreak, sings with the joys of seeing living things grow, with the love of my family, with the smiles of children. I am stronger in knowing I can't be taken advantage of again because I don't trust a soul.

If you don't trust anyone, you'll never get run over. Never be hurt. Never lose out.

July 20, 2018

Cogitation. Frustration. 100 years ago, Horace's mother was 2 years old. My grandmother was 12. My grandfather was 24. In a hundred years will anyone even remember me? Will anyone care enough to? If mother had lived, she would have been 83 in April this year. I took a flower to her grave site this year and I cried for the first time in a while. I didn't cry because I miss her (because technically, I don't) but because for the first time since I've been going to take her a flower, I didn't hear her anymore. I heard Mama and Papa (I always do). I even heard the faint Whispers of great grandma and Grandpa and great-great grandpa Jerry, but Mother's voice was gone.

Yes, I know I sound insane. It's okay to judge me. I get it all the time. I don't see the Dead (well, not often) or hear their voice with my ears (most of the time). Mostly it's a voice in my head that I know isn't mine.

Mother and I may have been close until my sister was born. But after that I was constantly trying to win everyone in my family's affection because they basically forgot about me when Melissa was born with colic. I even forgot about myself, as well, I suppose, because I fed her things she could stomach which were Foods that my little rotund ass loved, and never even sneaked a bite. Huge feat! For a three-year-old. And all the while, the "impressive child" (that was me), the child who has a cousin named after her because she was "so smart", the kid who wanted to be a doctor when she grew up (even at three years old) just faded into the background.

My grandmother still stood by me and saw me, somewhat. But there were times she was in another world, herself. When she did fight for me in some type of situation, the Thunder of their argument became almost as loud as the Thunder of the Dozen voices in my preteen head. So, I found a place to hide where only me and MY voices were, until their thunder stopped.

It was in that place I learned that many of the dark creatures or just like me. They were scared and alone. And if I didn't bother them, they left me be. So I would write and listen to a little portable radio I had. They spun their webs above

My Red curtain that I'd laid on the dirt where I hid. Under our Mill House, by an open vent, I could look out and see the front yard and part of the side yard, but no one knew I was there. I played my music just loud enough for me to hear, so it drowned out the thunder in my brain and my grandmother and mother arguing above me. And I wrote. They never knew I was there, and I wrote, and I wrote.

And within myself I was alone. I had friends, but I was still alone. Alone, because I couldn't tell them the huge gashes on my legs when I was 8 didn't come from my falling or from playing, but from sticking both legs under a rusty chicken wire fence and pulling back hard to see if that pain could make the pain inside go away for just a little while. And when it did (even for just a few days), I kept that on file for when the demons got unbearable again. As I write this now, I sit here, crying on the inside (because I can't cry on the outside) because I still feel all the pain that little girl felt. It was the first time I self-mutilated, but it would not be the last.

To say mother and I weren't close sounds horrible. I truly loved her. I still do. But I could never please her. I could never impress her or do good enough for her. I could never do anything she didn't criticize. My sister was perfect, and I was up a fuck-up. I grew up too fast. I walked too soon. I'm married too early. I was a horrible mother. To her, I was a disappointment. I couldn't even lose weight without her saying it was malnutrition or drugs (both of which never happened). Oh, unless it was from mother and my medical doctor putting me on black beauties in second grade. I lost weight on drugs they gave me.

To say I worshipped her? I don't know. I sometimes wish, when I see how close everyone else has been with their moms, how they take pictures smiling with Mom, Dad, and siblings, that I had had that.

My sister took my mother first, because she was so sick as a baby. Then she took my grandfather, because I was " too heavy to pick up anymore"(and it was right I was over a hundred pounds. But I was also 4 years old). Then, much later in life, I watched her take my grandmother. She couldn't take my favorite uncle who adored me, but he died when I was 10, so I had no one again. As an adult, she tried and failed to take my children. My mother even supported her at first. So, is it any wonder that mother and I aren't close? Oh! Excuse me! Weren't close. ☐

Why, after all of this, did I keep trying and trying to do good for her? Why did I keep pushing myself to things I knew that my fragile mental status would and could not handle? She was my mom. Regardless of whether she loved me or not, I loved her.

She thought I didn't need her because I was intelligent and mature for my age, but I needed a mother. I needed a father, too. The only man who ever really love me like a father and was proud of me like a dad should have been died when I was 10. My real dad hid from me. He never paid child support to my mother although they were married. He never acknowledged me as his daughter. When I found him at 30, he lied to me. And before he died at 66, he put every dime he had into a trust in his sons' names, so I'd never see a dime of it, even though I've never wanted money to begin with. I just wanted my family.

Turkey Buzzard   *Angela Luck*

Most days I am fine. I have my family now that are mine and they love me. Just when I remember old times and how I was made to feel, sometimes it all comes flooding back. All of the loneliness, sadness, and feelings of inadequacy surface and make my heart ache for normalcy. It can't happen.

It's the stuff my dreams would have been made of. If I was normal: which I'm not. And I never will be.

July 30, 2018

Someone who doesn't have a house doesn't see how upsetting it is when your yard and garden are going to hell because you don't feel like doing yard work. My yard is my joy. Right now, it's my shame, because it looks so bad. Once I get to feeling better, it'll going to be the talk of the neighborhood again! My joy and my pride, my peace and freedom are in my yard!

September 25, 2018

When I'm sick, all kinds of things go through my head. I enjoy having someone with me, but I hate being forced into things that I hate doing.

I know love is supposed to be give and take. Shouldn't I get something out of a relationship? Sometime? Somewhere?

It's at the point where all I do get is "I love you", and honestly, that's not enough. Saying is one thing but doing is another.

I'm tired, in almost constant pain, and so, so very alone.

What am I going to do next?

October 4, 2018

Ya know, I shouldn't still be obsessing about someone and something that happened over 2 years ago. But I am.

I shouldn't be trying to get an account back simply because it was mine to begin with. Because I set it up for him. But I am.

And it's so totally become my life's work until I get it done. Why?

I honestly have no idea whatsoever.

But I find myself waiting for the time when I can get back into Facebook, so I can try to get this account claimed back for myself again. I failed the first time. I won't mess up again. I'm going to delete all the friend requests and clear everything that needs to be cleared.

I have court in the morning. I'm not even phased by that.

All I can think about is getting control of this account again and getting part of the pics deleted and adding pics back that I think she got in and deleted off his profile when it was mine. Then I'll fix it to where she can't get back into that account again because I'll change the password to one that's so hard to guess, she'll never know what it is.

Turkey Buzzard *Angela Luck*

And I honestly still don't know why.

I guess what pisses me off so bad is the fact that I know she's been into the account messing. And I know it's MY account that I set up. I used it and I've been the only one who's had access to it.

That's just twisted. Something has to give. The best thing I can do it delete both accounts and let it be done. I know this, but I can't do it.

Somewhere in my life there has to be some kind of control. This is the only control I have left. And I just can't leave it hanging.

October 14, 2018

Other people are blessed.

Oh, I'm blessed, too, in the fact that I still can and do smile through everything I've been through all these years.

Let me explain: As I have transcribed these journals, a lot of the pain, mental anguish, and simple agony of being bipolar has flooded back into my person. I've had to fight with myself to keep from simply imploding and going off some mental deep end that is of my own making.

Other, more normal folk can let things go more easily. Death, I deal with fairly well on the whole, but abuse, both physical and mental, is a little harder to loosen the old fingers from around.

Having spoken to many other bipolar friends and acquaintances, I know it's a thorn in all our sides. It seems like we just can't let go of things as easily as other people. We tend to dwell on things more if they get brought back to surface.

In my years growing up, manic depression (bipolar disorder) wasn't understood as well as it is now. And it's still a mystery, because everyone has something in their make-up that is different and causes the beast to act differently when it attacks each individual who has it in another manner at times.

It makes treating this demon a lot harder for those who treat it. It makes dealing with it a lot harder for family, because even if they've dealt with another family member with it, it's not the same. It makes being a parent of a child with its hell. And it makes life for the person who has it a living hell sometimes as well, because it can change its stripes in midstream, too.

As I've dredged up these previous writings, though they've been quite recent (most of my previous journals have been destroyed by my own hand years ago), they still tend to drag me back into the time they were written. They bring back the feelings I was feeling when I wrote them. They sometimes even resurface the feelings of the events from long ago I was writing about.

When the final line is written on this first offering, my tumbled and jumbled mind is also already turning and tossing more writing for the second journal. The second book of this series.

This started out as a single book, but once I started writing, I knew there had to be more. There had to be not only an understanding of the things that made me into who I am, but also of how things have turned and turned in my life until I've become this person that I am now.

Trust me, I'm not perfect or complete. I'm still and probably always will be messed up beyond anybody's repair efforts, including my own. I've just managed to keep my outlook through a lot of prayer and a lot of feeling that I'm not totally sure where I'll end up in the next life, yet.

That being said, I think I'll leave those dalliances for another time.

Let's just say everything in my life remains conflicted. It's sad but true. I don't know why it's that way, but I do know that I keep doing things that I don't feel comfortable with in the long run. I keep condemning myself for things I've done in the past. And I keep hoping I can make amends for my wrongs in the future.

Turkey Buzzard *Angela Luck*

Oddly, this is where I've chosen to end this first foray into my own mind. Believe me when I say, there is more. There is so much more.

Through the urging of a few very instrumental cousins and friends, I decided to try publication of this journal and the musings of my tortured mind, in order to try to help others who have had similar circumstances and let them know they are not alone.

Let me continue by saying, I'd like to see others who haven't had any experience with bipolar or mental illness have an opportunity to read this and hopefully, the next book I'll be writing.

I am mentally ill. I feel more than others sometimes. I tend to hide it. I get hurt and I get mad and I rant and rave.

We are all human. Maybe you've seen something of yourself in this book. Maybe you haven't. I just hope somewhere you've felt something as you've read my words. I hope you've seen into my heart, even just a little.

And I hope you've enjoyed this. I've been writing since I was ten, hoping someday someone would read something I wrote and enjoy it or be touched by it.

Turkey Buzzard *Angela Luck*

Thanks to all who have read my words and continue to ride with me on my journey. I know it's a bumpy one, but if we manage to save just one small soul, then I'll feel that it's been worth the ride.

www.ingramcontent.com/pod-product-compliance
Lightning Source LLC
Chambersburg PA
CBHW020438220526
45464CB00002B/760